Monologue:

This book is dedicated to all the mothers and mother in-laws who have passed. When my mother in-law became ill and passed in hospice, we had no manual on what to do next as death quickly approached. We were scared and wanted to do the right thing and make the right choices in the right order. We wanted to make sure her legacy was fulfilled, and her spirit would live forever. We asked a hospice nurse at the time for a guide to help us along the way. We thought they would have a small paper book or a sheet of paper of steps to take to achieve our mother's honor. Instead, we were surprised that this was not available. Since then, I've been inspired to help others along this path like me so they can feel at ease in time of despair.

About the Author:

I grew up in Daytona Beach and used to take a school bus to church when I was 5. I have a beautiful family and we still go to the same church. A lot of my inspiration has always been spiritual. I'm an avid watermen and love to travel and watch sports. One of my fondest memories is when my mom took me to get cookies as a kid in Chicago. She always took care of our family and made sure we had everything we needed. If your mom is still alive give her a call and tell her, you love her. Thanks, mom, for always being the light in our lives.

Table of Contents

Chapter 1: The Knowledge of Death

Chapter 2: Planning the Funeral

Chapter 3: Caring for their Things

Chapter 4: The Death Certificate

Chapter 5: The Will

Chapter 6: Inventory of Assets

Chapter 7: Canceling Services

Chapter 8: The Social Presence

Chapter 9: A Show of Gratitude

Chapter 10: Distribution of Personal Belongings

Chapter 1: The Knowledge of Death

When the heart-wrenching news of a loved one's passing arrives, the initial steps must be taken with precision and compassion. This chapter delves into the practicalities that follow, guiding you through the first crucial moments of handling this profound loss.

1. The Pronouncement of Death: Obtaining a formal declaration of death is a necessary step to acquire the death certificate, which holds significant importance for legal proceedings and administrative matters. If the passing occurred within a medical facility, a qualified professional will handle the pronouncement. However, if it took place at home, contacting emergency services (911) is vital, and the deceased should be transferred to a medical facility for official confirmation.

2. Sharing the News of Loss: The burden of sharing this heartrending news with family, friends, and possibly an employer can feel overwhelming for one person. A suggested approach is to designate a few trusted individuals to shoulder this responsibility collectively. By dividing the task, each can support one another through the challenging process of conveying the solemn truth.

3. The Family Meeting: Coming together as a family is a fundamental aspect of navigating this difficult time. A family meeting provides an opportunity to discuss and respect the wishes of the departed regarding their funeral or memorial

arrangements, especially if they hadn't expressed their preferences before. Collaboratively deciding on a meaningful way to honor their memory helps bring closure and strengthens familial bonds.

In these initial moments of grief, knowledge and preparation are indispensable. By following these practical guidelines, you can navigate the complexities that arise after the passing of a loved one with clarity and compassion. Remember, though the journey may seem daunting, taking one step at a time will lead you towards a path of healing and remembrance.

Chapter 2: Planning the Funeral

As the weight of grief persists, practical matters demand attention. This chapter delves into the essential steps of planning a funeral, honoring the departed's wishes while navigating the financial aspects with care and consideration.

1. Seek Out Pertinent Documents: Before embarking on the funeral arrangements, it is prudent to scour the departed's personal effects for any relevant paperwork. Unearthed documents might reveal a prepaid burial plot, explicit cremation preferences, or financial provisions made in advance. By discovering such vital information, you can avoid unnecessary complications and align the funeral plans with the departed's heartfelt desires.

2. Compare Funeral Home Prices: In the midst of profound emotional turmoil, it is crucial to approach funeral planning with discernment. Taking the time to research and compare prices from various funeral homes enables the family to make informed decisions while ensuring that the chosen services align with both emotional and financial considerations. By exploring different options, you can create a meaningful and respectful farewell without undue financial strain.

3. Unveiling Veteran Benefits: For those who served their country, special considerations await. Families of veterans may qualify for funeral benefits, providing much-needed support during this difficult time. Delving into the available benefits and resources can alleviate financial burdens and bestow the respect and recognition our veterans deserve.

4. Embrace Family Support: The communal strength of family proves invaluable as the funeral planning unfolds. In an effort to lessen the financial load, family members can come together and pitch in. A collaborative approach allows loved ones to take on essential roles during the funeral, such as serving as pallbearers or assisting with various tasks. This shared responsibility fosters a sense of unity and devotion to honor the departed's memory in a heartfelt manner.

5. Personalizing the Farewell: Amid the practical considerations, don't overlook the power of personalization. Each life is a unique tapestry of experiences, and the funeral should reflect the individuality of the departed. Whether through cherished readings, beloved music, or heartfelt eulogies, incorporating personal touches creates a profound and lasting tribute to their life's journey.

Navigating the intricacies of funeral planning can be overwhelming, but with a methodical approach and the support of loved ones, it becomes a tribute of profound significance. As each step is taken with care, the funeral takes shape as a testament of love and reverence, embodying the essence of the one who has departed. In the embrace of family, the departed's legacy is celebrated, providing solace and healing to all who gather to honor their memory.

Chapter 3: Caring for their Things

Amidst the tumult of funeral preparations, tending to the practical aspects of the departed's life becomes a pressing necessity. This chapter offers guidance on how to care for their belongings, secure their home, and ensure the well-being of their pets, all while providing some breathing room to cope with the grieving process.

1. Safeguarding the Home: As the heartbeat of memories, the departed's home holds both sentimental and practical value. To safeguard the property and its cherished possessions, family members should take immediate steps to secure it. Locking doors and windows provides a sense of reassurance, while ensuring that personal valuables like jewelry find temporary refuge in a secure safety deposit box preserves their integrity until a permanent plan is determined.

2. Tending to Beloved Pets: If pets were a cherished part of the departed's life, making provisions for their well-being becomes an essential consideration. Family members can come together to discuss and decide who among them can provide a loving home for these faithful companions. Alternatively, exploring reputable adoption centers or fostering programs allows for a compassionate transition of care, ensuring that these beloved animals find the comfort and care they deserve.

3. Managing Mail Matters: Addressing the practicalities of daily life is crucial during this delicate period. To prevent mail from

accumulating and adding to the weight of emotions, it is advisable to arrange for mail forwarding from the deceased's address to a designated family member's home. Additionally, notifying magazines and other marketing entities to halt subscriptions prevents unnecessary reminders of the departed's absence, offering a small measure of relief in an otherwise challenging time.

4. Tackling Essential Tasks: While larger decisions may take time, smaller essential tasks must not be overlooked. Paying outstanding bills, canceling services that are no longer needed, and informing relevant institutions of the passing will help streamline matters in the days to come. Family members can work together to ensure these tasks are addressed efficiently and with the care they deserve.

5. Allowing Space for Reflection: Amidst the practicalities, it is crucial to grant yourself and your family members the space to process emotions and mourn your loss. Balancing the necessary tasks with personal well-being can be challenging, but by supporting one another and taking each step with compassion, the burden becomes lighter to bear.

In the intricate dance of caring for their belongings, pets, and mail, a delicate balance emerges between practicality and emotion. In preserving their home and possessions, attending to their pets, and managing everyday affairs, you continue to honor their memory. Through this shared responsibility, the departed's life finds a tender continuity, while you, their cherished family, find strength and resilience in the unity of care.

Chapter 4: The Death Certificate

In the wake of a loved one's passing, the death certificate emerges as a pivotal document, essential for managing their assets and end-of-life affairs. This chapter delves into the significance of the death certificate, its content, and the necessary steps to obtain this crucial record.

1. Understanding the Death Certificate: The death certificate is a legal document that serves as an official record of a person's passing. Signed by a licensed medical professional, it contains vital information about the deceased, including their full name, date of birth, date of death, and other identifying details. Additionally, the certificate includes pertinent data concerning the cause of death, an important aspect for official documentation.

2. The Significance of the Death Certificate: Recognizing the pivotal role of the death certificate in the aftermath of a loss is crucial. This document acts as a gateway to the deceased's assets and financial affairs. To facilitate the proper handling of end-of-life matters, obtaining multiple copies of the death certificate is advisable. Approximately 10-12 copies are typically required when dealing with tasks such as closing bank accounts, managing brokerage accounts, and settling insurance claims.

3. Who Can Obtain the Death Certificate: Understanding who is eligible to obtain a copy of the death certificate is essential. Checking with your city or county clerk's office ensures clarity

on the process. Generally, close relatives of the deceased, such as spouses, children, or parents, can request a copy by providing proper proof of identity and payment. This verification safeguards the confidentiality and security of this sensitive information.

4. Certified or Non-Certified: Death certificates come in two forms—certified and non-certified. Certified copies hold official standing and are required for most legal and financial matters. Non-certified copies, while still containing relevant information, are typically used for informational purposes only. Depending on the nature of the affairs to be handled, ensuring you have an adequate number of certified copies is essential.

5. Navigating with Care: Dealing with the death certificate is a sensitive and critical task. It is crucial to approach this process with utmost care and attention to detail. Collaborating with the proper authorities, such as the medical practitioner, local officials, or a funeral director, helps ensure the accuracy and validity of the document. By navigating this step thoughtfully, you set the foundation for effectively managing your departed loved one's assets and finalizing their affairs.

As the gateway to administering the deceased's financial and personal matters, the death certificate plays an integral role in the aftermath of loss. With a clear understanding of its significance and proper procedures, you can approach this process with confidence and alleviate future complications. May this essential document serve as a catalyst for a smooth transition, enabling you to honor the memory of your loved one with clarity and grace.

Chapter 5: The Will

Within the realm of fulfilling the final wishes of the departed lies the power of the will—an instrumental document that paves the way for a smooth and purposeful distribution of assets. This chapter delves into the crucial steps involved in honoring the deceased's intentions, beginning with the quest to locate the will and its designated executor.

1. Unearthing the Will and Executor: The journey of executing a will begins with a meticulous search for the document itself. From desks to safety lockboxes, and wherever the departed might have stored essential papers, every nook must be explored to discover this vital legal testament. Once found, the will often designates an executor—the person entrusted with the responsibility of carrying out the deceased's final wishes. In cases where no executor is named, the court will appoint an administrator to fulfill this pivotal role.

2. Enlisting the Aid of Trust and Estates Attorney: For estates valued at over $50,000, navigating the legal intricacies of asset management requires the expertise of a trust and estates attorney. These knowledgeable professionals provide essential guidance in ensuring that the distribution of assets aligns with the legal requirements of the state. To ensure a seamless process, it is crucial to familiarize yourself with the laws and regulations governing estate distribution in your particular jurisdiction.

3. Discovering and Assessing All Assets: As the journey of managing the estate unfolds, the task of identifying all the assets of the departed takes center stage. From real estate and financial holdings to personal belongings of sentimental value, each asset must be accounted for. Through meticulous record-keeping and collaborative efforts, you can ensure that nothing of significance is overlooked.

4. Initiation of Probate: Once the will has been located and the executor or administrator identified, the legal process of probate begins. Probate is the formal validation of the will by the court, confirming its authenticity and providing the legal authority to distribute the assets according to the deceased's wishes. This essential step marks the commencement of the journey to fulfill the departed's bequests.

5. Navigating with Sensitivity and Diligence: The handling of the will and estate distribution requires both sensitivity and diligence. Throughout this process, emotions run high, and the gravity of responsibilities must be met with care. By enlisting the assistance of experienced legal professionals, you can navigate these complexities with poise and respect, ensuring that the legacy of the departed is preserved in a manner befitting their intentions.

In the pursuit of executing the will, you embark on a journey guided by the vision of the departed. As you uncover and uphold the wishes they left behind, may the process be one of unity and understanding, allowing the memory of your loved one to shine brightly through the fulfillment of their legacy.

Chapter 6: Inventory of Assets

In the aftermath of loss, the task of inventorying the deceased's assets emerges, akin to a meticulous scavenger hunt that requires diligence and attention to detail. This chapter outlines essential steps in this process, ensuring a comprehensive account of all assets to facilitate their distribution in accordance with the will.

1. Unraveling the Assets: The journey of locating the deceased's assets can indeed feel like embarking on a complex scavenger hunt. From real estate and financial accounts to valuable heirlooms, every valuable item holds significance in the inheritance puzzle. To navigate this process efficiently, consider seeking the expertise of professional asset location services, which can assist in uncovering all aspects of the estate for a nominal fee.

2. Crafting a Comprehensive List: Once each asset is unearthed, a comprehensive inventory should be meticulously crafted. This list becomes a crucial record, ensuring that nothing is overlooked or omitted. The compiled inventory should be entrusted to the appropriate individual, typically the executor, to be accurately filed for future reference.

3. Addressing Financial Obligations: Alongside asset discovery, it is essential to gather all of the deceased's bills and financial obligations. Whether utility payments, outstanding loans, or other financial commitments, compiling an inclusive list ensures that these matters can be addressed appropriately. The executor plays a pivotal role in finalizing these bills, ensuring that the estate's resources are allocated efficiently.

4. Empowering the Executor: The executor takes center stage in this process, carrying the weight of managing and distributing the deceased's assets. Equipped with the comprehensive inventory and bill list, the executor navigates this responsibility with prudence and accuracy, honoring the departed's intentions and preserving the estate's integrity.

5. The Legacy of Care: The inventory of assets is a testament to the value and impact the departed's life had on those around them. As you meticulously compile this record, you continue to honor their memory and uphold their legacy of careful planning and provision for their loved ones. Through the clarity and thoroughness of this inventory, the final wishes of the departed find expression, weaving a legacy of compassion and foresight.

In the process of inventorying assets, you embark on a journey that embraces the intricacies of a life well-lived. Through the collaborative efforts of the executor and the support of those involved, the legacy of your loved one is upheld with respect and diligence. May this chapter be a guiding light in the careful administration of the estate, ensuring that the essence of the departed endures for generations to come.

Chapter 7: Canceling Services

In the intricate process of tying up loose ends, this chapter offers guidance on canceling services utilized by the departed. Approach this task with organization and care, ensuring that each service is addressed thoroughly to honor the departed's memory and financial affairs.

1. Compilation of Service List: As the family navigates the aftermath of loss, designating someone to meticulously comb through the deceased's mail, files, and drawers is essential. By creating a comprehensive list of all services used by the departed, you lay the groundwork for a systematic approach to canceling each one.

2. Ceasing General Services: With the list of services in hand, it falls upon the family to initiate the process of cancelation. Contacting each service provider individually, the responsible family member should communicate the news of the passing and request the termination of the respective service. Some companies may require a copy of the death certificate before taking any action. The persistence of compassion and understanding during these calls fosters a smooth transition in the cessation of these services.

3. Attending to Identity Accounts: In the meticulous process of cancelation, it is crucial not to overlook personal accounts

associated with the deceased's identity. From their driver's license to social security, life insurance policies, and other personal accounts, each entity should be notified of the passing and provided with the necessary documentation, such as a copy of the death certificate, to complete the cancelation process. Ensuring that each of these accounts is responsibly and thoroughly addressed brings closure to this chapter of the family's journey.

4. The Journey of Letting Go: Canceling services is a poignant chapter in the journey of letting go. As you approach each task with respect and efficiency, you honor the departed's legacy and attend to the practicalities that reflect their life's journey. Through this process, the memory of your loved one remains embedded in the conscientious administration of their affairs, each cancelation an act of love and responsibility.

5. Supporting One Another: Throughout this phase, emotions may surface, making it essential to support one another with kindness and empathy. By sharing the responsibilities and maintaining open lines of communication, the burden becomes lighter to bear, fostering unity and solidarity among family members.

As you traverse this chapter of canceling services, know that you are tending to your loved one's legacy with diligence and care. Each service canceled is a step towards closure, honoring the memory of the departed while setting the stage for the next phase of the journey. Together, you navigate this process, ensuring that your loved one's life is celebrated in each act of responsibility and remembrance.

Chapter 8: The Social Presence

In the era of social media and online connectivity, managing the digital footprint of the deceased becomes a crucial task. This chapter sheds light on options for handling their social media accounts and the importance of closing other online accounts, ensuring the protection of their digital legacy.

1. Care of Social Media Accounts: When it comes to social media accounts, families have options to consider. Some may choose to close the deceased's accounts entirely, while others opt to "memorialize" them. Memorializing a social media account allows it to remain as a tribute, preserving the memories and allowing friends and loved ones to post on the departed's timeline. Understanding the platform's policies and guidelines regarding memorialization helps navigate this sensitive decision.

2. Closing Email Accounts: Email accounts hold a wealth of personal information, making it crucial to address their closure. Leaving email accounts active can pose a risk of identity theft or unauthorized access. Take the necessary steps to close the deceased's email accounts, ensuring the privacy and security of their digital correspondence. Remember to verify if the deceased had multiple email accounts to address each one appropriately.

3. Managing Other Online Accounts: Beyond social media and email, it is essential to consider other online accounts the deceased may have had. These can include platforms such as PayPal, survey companies that payout funds, or training sites they were registered with. Take the time to identify and close these accounts, ensuring that any remaining funds or credits are appropriately disbursed. In some cases, you may need to provide proof of identity, along with a copy of the death certificate, to facilitate the closure process.

4. Preserving Digital Legacy: Each step taken to manage the deceased's online presence contributes to the preservation of their digital legacy. By carefully considering how to handle social media accounts and closing online platforms, you honor their memory and protect their privacy. While these actions may seem technical in nature, they carry emotional weight, reflecting the care and respect you have for the departed.

5. Nurturing Memories: As you navigate the digital realm, remember that it is just one facet of the rich tapestry of memories left behind. While tending to online accounts is necessary, it is equally important to nurture and cherish the tangible memories shared with your loved one. Through the interplay of the physical and digital, the legacy of the departed lives on, illuminating the lives they touched.

In the chapter of closing memories, the management of the deceased's social presence plays a pivotal role. By thoughtfully addressing social media accounts, email closures, and other online platforms, you safeguard their digital legacy and honor their online presence. As you navigate this delicate terrain, may it serve as a means to celebrate the cherished memories that endure in the hearts and minds of all who loved them.

Chapter 9: A Show of Gratitude

In the midst of the whirlwind that follows the passing of a family member, it is common for expressions of gratitude to take a back seat. However, as life begins to settle, finding moments to acknowledge those who provided emotional support and offered their blessings and gifts becomes a meaningful endeavor. This chapter explores various ways to show gratitude to those who have been there during this challenging time.

1. Arrange a Heartfelt Visit: For those who are physically close, arranging a visit to sit and talk can be one of the most meaningful ways to show your appreciation. Sharing moments together, reminiscing, and expressing gratitude in person allow for a deeper connection and an opportunity to convey the sincerity of your feelings.

2. Cards of Acknowledgement: For loved ones who are geographically distant but have offered their support from afar, sending thoughtful cards of acknowledgement is a heartfelt gesture. Taking the time to express your gratitude in writing demonstrates the depth of your appreciation for their presence during this challenging period.

3. Embrace Technology for Connection: In this age of advanced communication, technology offers various means of connecting with others regardless of distance. Facetime, video chat, and texting are excellent options to express your thanks to those who have been there for you. The beauty of technology lies in its ability to bridge the gap and create a sense of closeness even across vast distances.

4. A Moment of Reflection: In dedicating time for gratitude, you create a moment of reflection and appreciation for all the support received. Whether through personal visits, cards, or digital connections, your expression of gratitude serves not only as a testament to your loved one's impact on your life but also as a testament to the strength of your relationships.

5. An Exchange of Love: As you extend your gratitude to those who have been by your side, you engage in a beautiful exchange of love and support. This act of reciprocity fosters deeper bonds with those who have offered solace, and it becomes a collective journey of healing and connection.

In the chapter of showing gratitude, the richness of human connections shines through. Through heartfelt visits, thoughtful cards, or virtual conversations, you communicate the profound impact that others' support has had on your journey. By nurturing these relationships, you not only honor the memory of your departed loved one but also forge a lasting sense of community and love that sustains you through the healing process.

Chapter 10: Distribution of Personal Belongings

In the poignant chapter of distributing the deceased's personal belongings, emotions run deep, and cherished memories come to the forefront. This chapter offers insights and advice on navigating this delicate process, acknowledging the role of the executor, honoring memory keepsakes, and managing family tensions with empathy and grace.

1. The Executor's Role: As the entrusted executor, the individual takes on the weighty responsibility of sorting through the departed's personal items. This entails making decisions about donations, sales, and the distribution of belongings. Recognizing the emotional significance of each possession, the executor may seek the family's assistance in deciding how to handle particular items, fostering a sense of unity and collaboration.

2. Memory Keepsakes: In the time leading up to their passing, the deceased may have expressed their desire for specific items to be given to certain individuals as cherished keepsakes. These memory treasures are imbued with sentimental value, and it is essential for the family to come together and respect and acknowledge these wishes as much as possible.

3. Navigating Family Tensions: The passing of a loved one can evoke complex emotions, leading to tension among family members during the distribution process. Recognizing the potential for disagreements, it is crucial to approach the situation with patience and empathy. The goal is not to ensure everyone's happiness, but rather to put the memories shared with the deceased into perspective and honor their legacy with mutual respect.

4. An Embrace of Healing: In the distribution of personal belongings, you embark on a journey of healing, preserving the essence of the departed and nurturing the relationships among the living. By fostering open communication and understanding, you create an atmosphere of compassion that allows emotions to find expression and healing to take root.

5. Holding onto Treasured Memories: Amidst the distribution, it is essential to remember that the true legacy of your loved one lies not only in their possessions but in the memories shared and the love they brought into your life. Each item may hold sentimental value, but the true treasure resides in the heartfelt connections that endure beyond material possessions.

As you navigate the chapter of distribution, remember that it is a journey of both farewells and celebrations. By honoring memory keepsakes, managing family tensions, and holding onto treasured memories, you create a space where healing can flourish. In the collective embrace of your loved one's legacy, you find strength and unity as a family, forging bonds that endure and celebrating a life well-lived.

Notes:

Notes

Notes

Notes

Made in the USA
Columbia, SC
31 July 2023